MASTERING MINIMALISM

MASTERING MINIMALISM

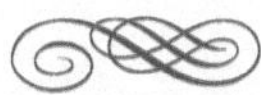

*Declutter Your Way to
a Simpler Life*

B. VINCENT

QuantumQuill Press

Contents

1   Chapter 1: Understanding Minimalism   1

2   Chapter 2: Assessing Your Current Situation   8

3   Chapter 3: The Art of Decluttering   15

4   Chapter 4: Simplifying Your Digital Life   23

5   Chapter 5: Minimalist Living Spaces   30

6   Chapter 6: Cultivating Minimalist Habits   37

7   Chapter 7: Minimalism Beyond Material Possessions   44

8   Chapter 8: Overcoming Challenges and Embracing Growth   52

9   Conclusion: Living a Fulfilling Minimalist Life   59

I

Chapter 1: Understanding Minimalism

The Explanation of Minimalism

Beyond mere emptiness and austere aesthetics, minimalism encompasses a profound philosophical stance that questions established beliefs regarding prosperity, contentment, and material success. Fundamentally, minimalism entails the process of eliminating extraneous elements in order to reveal what is genuinely significant in one's life. Deliberately reducing distractions and prioritizing the essential is a conscious decision that impairs our capacity to lead lives filled with intention and purpose.

Fundamentally, minimalism constitutes a state of mind—a deliberate choice to streamline one's existence through the elimination of mental and emotional burdens as well as material possessions. It pertains to adopting the liberation that results from relinquishing superfluous obligations and placing experiences above the accumulation of material possessions.

Establishing a definition for minimalism paves the way for an enlightening and profound voyage toward a more straightforward and gratifying life. This expedition prompts individuals to reassess their priorities, redefine their connection to consumerism, and develop a more profound appreciation for the abundance that can be discovered in the ordinary occurrences of existence.

The Historical Setting

In order to acquire a comprehensive understanding of minimalism, one must delve into its historical origins and comprehend the cultural and philosophical currents that have influenced its progressive development. Although minimalism may appear to be a modern phenomenon, its roots can be identified in ancient times and encompass a wide range of artistic movements and cultures.

Minimalism arose within the domains of art and design as a response to the extravagant embellishments that characterized the late 19th and early 20th centuries. Architects and artists endeavored to eliminate embellishments and frilly, placing a premium on light, space, and geometric shapes. Prominent individuals such as Ludwig Mies van der Rohe, Donald Judd, and the Bauhaus pioneers established the foundation for minimalist aesthetics by advocating for functionality and simplicity as defining characteristics of excellent design.

Minimalism, which extended beyond the domain of art, manifested itself in a multitude of philosophical and spiritual traditions. Minimalism, spanning from the Stoic philosophy's emphasis on interior tranquility in the face of external chaos to Zen Buddhism's emphasis on simplicity and mindfulness, shares enduring principles that advocate for living with intention and integrity.

Understanding the historical backdrop of minimalism enables one to develop a more profound admiration for its enduring significance and immutable allure. This statement underscores the enduring philosophical nature of minimalism, which appeals to the fundamental human desire for simplicity, harmony, and significance in a world that is becoming progressively more intricate.

Positive Aspects of Minimalism

Minimalism provides an extensive array of advantages that transcend the surface-level allure of orderly areas and decluttered dwellings. Minimalism, at its essence, promotes deliberate and purposeful living—making informed decisions to prioritize what is genuinely essential and removing extraneous elements that diminish our overall state of being. Many facets of an individual's life can undergo profound changes through the adoption of minimalism.

One of the most notable advantages of minimalism is the tranquility and mental acuity that results from the cleansing of our physical environment. By streamlining our living spaces, we concurrently alleviate tension and frustration by decluttering our thoughts. This enhanced awareness enables us to direct our efforts and consideration towards the matters that genuinely require it, thereby cultivating a heightened sense of direction and satisfaction.

Additionally, by encouraging us to live within our means and avoid the pitfall of consumerism, minimalism fosters financial independence. We can cultivate a healthier relationship with money, reduce debt, and save money by prioritizing experiences over material possessions and avoiding superfluous purchases. We are able to pursue our pursuits, invest in meaningful experiences, and live life on our own terms due to this financial stability.

Conversely, by encouraging us to place relationships and experiences above material possessions, minimalism fosters more profound connections with others. We can spend more time and effort cultivating significant relationships with family, friends, and the community if we relinquish the pursuit of material wealth and social standing. Sincere connections of this nature enhance the quality of life and furnish us with encouragement and contentment that transcend the transient gratification of material possessions.

Furthermore, apart from the aforementioned concrete advantages, minimalism carries significant ramifications for our holistic welfare and contentment. The act of streamlining our lives and removing superfluous elements makes room for happiness, innovation, and individual development. It is ascertained that genuine pleasure is not found in the amassing of material goods, but rather in the instances of connection, intention, and appreciation that characterize a life filled with depth and significance.

In brief, minimalism offers extensive and diverse advantages, including enhancements to one's financial stability, mental health, and interpersonal connections. We can cultivate a more straightforward and purposeful lifestyle that results in increased satisfaction, joy, and tranquility by adopting minimalism.

Frequent Misconceptions

In popular culture, minimalism is frequently misrepresented and misconstrued, despite its increasing popularity. There are numerous misconceptions that perpetuate falsehoods, which could discourage individuals from diving into this life-altering way of life. By addressing these prevalent fallacies, we can enhance our comprehension of the true essence of minimalism and the advantages it can provide.

A widely held fallacy is the conviction that minimalism necessitates extreme austerity or deprivation. In opposition to this belief, minimalism does not entail reducing one's possessions to the minimum necessities or forgoing comfort and convenience. Conversely, the emphasis should be on deliberate existence and conscientious consumption—placing experiences above material possessions and prioritizing quality over quantity. Finding the optimal equilibrium that permits us to live comfortably while minimizing waste and excess is the essence of minimalism.

The misconception that minimalism is equivalent to renunciation of worldly indulgences or asceticism is another prevalent one. Although certain individuals may select to embrace a minimalist way of life as a means of spiritual devotion, minimalism does not possess an intrinsic association with any specific religious or philosophical worldview. Minimalism is a versatile philosophy that can be modified to accommodate personal inclinations and situations, enabling each individual to establish its own definition.

Moreover, the simplistic approach is frequently depicted as a universal remedy, which may misinform individuals into thinking that it is exclusively appropriate for particular personality types or ways of life. Minimalism is, in actuality, a profoundly individual endeavor, and there is no singular "correct" method of its application. Minimalism can be adapted to suit the specific requirements and preferences of individuals residing in rural areas or in the city, including active professionals who must contend with urban bustle.

Ultimately, minimalism is occasionally disregarded as a transitory fashion or way of life phenomenon, devoid of substantiality or enduring influence. Nevertheless, mindfulness, intentionality, and simplicity—the tenets of minimalism—have been adopted by philosophies and cultures alike over the course of time. Minimalism is an enduring philosophy that provides advice and direction for navigating the complexities of contemporary life; it is not a passing fad.

By rectifying these prevalent misunderstandings, we can establish a foundation for a more sophisticated comprehension of minimalism and its capacity to enrich our existence in substantial and significant ways. The concept of minimalism does not entail strict adherence to rules or the compromise of comfort and pleasure. Rather, it advocates for a more deliberate and straightforward lifestyle that enables us to concentrate on what is truly essential.

Living a Minimalist Way of Life

In addition to the straightforward practice of organizing and decluttering our physical environments, minimalism incorporates a more comprehensive philosophy—a way of life—that permeates all facets of our being. Embracing minimalism entails embracing a mentality characterized by intentionality, mindfulness, and simplicity in all that we do.

Fundamentally, minimalism urges individuals to critically examine the ubiquity of consumerism in society and to reassess their connection to material possessions. This perspective questions the belief that happiness and satisfaction are contingent upon material possessions, and instead encourages us to discover contentment in the depths of experiences, interpersonal connections, and individual development.

The minimalist way of life promotes greater deliberateness and compels us to make decisions that are in accordance with our personal values and priorities. We create space in our lives for what truly matters by eliminating distractions and unnecessary items; this enables us to devote our time, energy, and resources to endeavors that bring us happiness, satisfaction, and significance.

Furthermore, minimalism cultivates a more profound state of mindfulness—an increased consciousness of the current moment and a recognition of the magnificence and plenty that envelop us. We learn to appreciate the beauty of the mundane, appreciate gratitude for the basic pleasures, and appreciate the richness of every moment by incorporating mindfulness into our daily lives.

A voyage, not a destination, minimalism entails an ongoing process of development and refinement. It urges us to consistently re-evaluate our priorities, eliminate superfluous matters, and endeavor to achieve enhanced simplicity and lucidity across all facets of our existence. By consistently engaging in this practice, we come to understand that genuine abundance is not found in the amassing of material goods, but rather in the liberation and satisfaction that ensue from living with a smaller amount.

Minimalism is, at its core, a philosophical stance that advocates for liberation, authenticity, and personal satisfaction. By adopting minimalism as a way of life, one can foster a more profound sense of purpose, connection, and pleasure, thereby transitioning to a more straightforward and significant way of being.

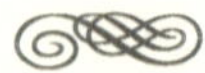

Chapter 2: Assessing Your Current Situation

Considerable Self-Reflection

Prior to commencing the process of streamlining and simplifying our lives through decluttering, it is critical to engage in some introspection and self-analysis. This procedure entails engaging in introspection and candidly evaluating our present state of affairs regarding possessions, disarray, and overall life contentment.

Initiating self-reflection entails posing introspective inquiries to oneself concerning one's consumption patterns, emotional investment in material possessions, and the day-to-day repercussions of congestion. Is it true that we frequently acquire new items in search of momentary gratification with each subsequent purchase? Do our disorganized and congested living spaces contribute to our anxiety and stress? And finally, are we genuinely satisfied with the manner in which we are conducting our daily lives?

Through the active pursuit of self-reflection, we acquire

significant understandings regarding the fundamental incentives that propel our actions as well as the domains of our lives that might require modification. This presents an occasion to confront any unease or discontent that we might be experiencing and to discern domains in which we can effectuate constructive modifications.

Additionally, through self-reflection, we can clarify our intentions and objectives in our pursuit of minimalism. Are we striving to imbue our lives with greater clarity and simplicity? Do we wish for additional leisure and autonomy to pursue our interests and passions? A comprehension of our motivations can assist us in maintaining concentration and dedication to our endeavor of decluttering, notwithstanding obstacles or setbacks.

Fundamentally, engaging in self-reflection signifies the initial stride towards adopting a more deliberate and uncomplicated lifestyle. We lay the groundwork for significant life transformation and change by engaging in introspection and a sincere evaluation of our present circumstances.

Recognizing Clutter

The process of identifying clutter extends beyond mere recognition of tangible accumulations of belongings; it necessitates comprehension of the diverse manifestations clutter can assume as well as its ramifications on our holistic welfare. Clutter extends beyond the realm of the physical, influencing the realm of the mind and emotions and engendering sentiments of discontentment, anxiety, and overwhelm.

Clutter can manifest in various ways within our physical environments, including stacked, unused items, overflowing closets, and congested countertops. It is critical to understand that debris pertains not only to an excessive quantity of possessions, but also to items that have outlived their usefulness or failed to add value to our existence. Commencing the process of decluttering and establishing a more tranquil and functional living space is possible when the origins of physical congestion in our residences are identified.

Nevertheless, the presence of disorder extends beyond the tangible environment and can manifest in the mental and emotional spheres as well. Mental congestion can manifest as a preoccupation with racing thoughts, persistent anxiety, or an incapacity to concentrate as a result of an overpowering sense of disorder. Conversely, emotional clutter can present itself in the form of unresolved emotions, detrimental interpersonal connections, or a sensation of being overburdened by negative sentiments.

To address congestion in all its forms in an effective manner, it is necessary to cultivate mindfulness and awareness of one's surroundings, thoughts, and emotions. By assessing the physical and mental congestion in our lives, we can initiate the process of recognizing recurring patterns and routines that could potentially be the source of our feelings of being inundated. This state of consciousness establishes the foundation for deliberately selecting options that optimize and simplify our existence, liberating ourselves from the weight of surplus and generating area for enhanced tranquility and lucidity.

Evaluating Priorities

It is effortless to become disoriented from our fundamental values amidst the disorderliness of contemporary existence. The process of prioritization assessment entails a moment of introspection regarding our fundamental principles and ambitions, which aids in the clarification of our desired life priorities.

It helps to commence this process by considering what brings us the most happiness and satisfaction. Do we prioritize spending quality time with our loved ones, pursuing our creative pursuits, or positively impacting our communities? We can begin to ascertain our true priorities by identifying the experiences and activities that touch us the most profoundly.

We can then assess the degree to which our present way of life corresponds with these values. Do we allocate our time and effort towards endeavors that align with our values and objectives, or do we become engrossed in pursuits that divert our attention from what is genuinely significant? Evaluating our daily rituals and habits can unveil instances in which we are deviating from our intended course of action, thereby furnishing invaluable discernment for rectification.

Additionally, we must consider the consequences of our decisions and actions in the long run. What kind of legacy do we wish to establish? What sort of influence do we wish to exert on the global community? By formulating objectives that are congruent with our priorities and imagining an optimal future, we can establish a strategic blueprint for leading a life that is more deliberate and purposeful.

The evaluation of priorities is a perpetual undertaking—a sustained voyage of introspection and improvement. We may find that our priorities change as we mature and develop, necessitating that we reevaluate and realign our lives on a consistent basis. Through maintaining an awareness of our deepest values and interests, we can foster an increased sense of contentment and fulfillment, which in turn contributes to a more significant and goal-oriented life.

Setting Objectives

After evaluating our priorities and attaining a clear understanding of what is genuinely significant to us, the subsequent course of action is to convert this comprehension into practical objectives. By providing a road map for our decluttering voyage, goal setting enables us to remain motivated and focused as we strive to create a more deliberate and uncomplicated existence.

It is critical to ensure that objectives are SMART (specific, measurable, achievable, pertinent, and time-bound) when establishing them. Increasing the likelihood of success, this guarantees that our objectives are explicit and executable. One possible illustration is to replace an imprecise objective like "decluttering my home" with a SMART goal: "over the course of the next month, organize one closet at a time."

Our objectives should, apart from being SMART, also correspond with our core values and priorities. By maintaining a clear vision of our lives in mind, we can guarantee that our objectives are significant and consistent with our overarching aspirations. This convergence enhances our drive and dedication to attaining our objectives, notwithstanding the challenges or setbacks that may arise.

Additionally, larger objectives can be simplified into more manageable duties. This facilitates a sense of confidence and enables us to commemorate advancements throughout the process. As an illustration, in the pursuit of completely decluttering our residence, we might partition this objective into more manageable components— e.g., tackling a specific category of items (e.g., books, apparel) or decluttering a single room.

Lastly, it is critical to review and modify our objectives on a regular basis. As circumstances are subject to change over time, life is a malleable entity that demands that we modify our plans accordingly. As we continue on our journey to declutter, we can ensure that our objectives remain pertinent and significant by remaining adaptable and receptive to new possibilities.

By establishing objectives, we can effectively manifest our aspirations into tangible outcomes. We can truly progress toward the creation of the simpler, more purposeful existence that we seek by establishing precise goals and implementing purposeful measures to attain them.

Comprehension of Resistance

It is not uncommon to face resistance along the path to decluttering and simplifying our lives; these are internal barriers and obstacles that impede our advancement. It is critical to comprehend and confront this resistance in order to surmount obstacles and maintain our dedication to the objective of decluttering.

Obstacles to progressing include procrastination, self-doubt, and aversion to change. We might discover that in order to avoid decluttering duties or justify the retention of particular possessions, we find ourselves making excuses. Frequently, these resistance patterns originate from profoundly entrenched routines and convictions concerning our possessions and our personal identity.

In order to surmount resistance, it is imperative to initially recognize and embrace the unease that it engenders. Feeling hesitant or uncertain is normal during the decluttering process; resistance is an expected consequence. By embracing our emotions without passing judgment, we can foster an environment conducive to self-compassion and comprehension, thereby enabling us to progress with enhanced clarity and determination.

Following this, it is beneficial to determine the fundamental causes of our resistance. Do we cling to our possessions out of security concerns, sentimental attachment, or dread of scarcity? We can start to challenge and reframe the limiting beliefs that may be impeding our progress by investigating the underlying causes of our resistance.

By identifying the origin of our resistance, we can subsequently devise effective strategies to overcome it. This may entail delegating responsibilities into more feasible components, seeking assistance from loved ones or friends, or engaging in self-care activities to alleviate anxiety and tension. By addressing our resistance proactively, we can gain confidence and impetus in our capacity to simplify and declutter our lives.

Ultimately, it is critical to commemorate our advancements and achievements throughout the process. Every incremental achievement advances our dedication to achieving our decluttering objectives and strengthens our resolve to live a more minimalistic and purposeful existence. By recognizing and commemorating our accomplishments, we can sustain our drive and inspiration to further our decluttering endeavors, surmount opposition, and wholeheartedly embrace the paradigm-shifting potential of minimalism.

3

Chapter 3: The Art of Decluttering

Commencing Our Work

Beginning the process of decluttering can be a daunting endeavor, particularly when confronted with the insurmountable challenge of sifting through a lifetime's worth of accumulated belongings. However, starting is an essential initial action that must be taken in order to achieve success.

Initiating the decluttering process with a well-defined strategy can be beneficial. Determine a particular area or category of belongings—such as a disorganized kitchen larder, cluttered closet, or overflowing bookshelf—to address initially. Facilitating the decluttering process by dividing it into smaller, more feasible tasks can enhance its accessibility and prevent feelings of being overwhelming.

After determining a starting point, schedule specific time to concentrate on decluttering. Consistency is essential, whether it be a few minutes each day or a few hours over the weekend. Establish a lifestyle-compatible decluttering schedule and make it a point to adhere to it; decluttering should be regarded as a top priority, not an afterthought.

Start the process of decluttering with an attitude of inquisitiveness and investigation. When evaluating each item, adopt a discerning mindset and inquire of yourself, "Does this item fulfill a specific function in my life?" Does it contribute in any way to my happiness or worth? If the response is negative, it might be appropriate to relinquish the situation.

Bear in mind that the objective of decluttering is not perfection, but rather advancement. Maintain a loving attitude toward yourself and commemorate incremental triumphs throughout the process. Accomplishing even the most modest task of organizing an entire room or a single compartment signifies progress toward the overarching objective of leading a more deliberate and uncomplicated existence.

Commencing the process of decluttering signifies an initial stride towards establishing an environment that mirrors one's personal values and priorities. Having an open mind and a readiness to relinquish, embrace the process with the understanding that the release of each item makes way for increased tranquility, independence, and clarity in your existence.

Room-by-Room Methodology

The task of decluttering can be daunting when one is confronted with the totality of their living area. Hence, by employing a room-by-room methodology, one can methodically and systematically approach the task at hand, thereby rendering it more feasible and less intimidating.

Select a room, preferable one that is less overwhelming or where the clutter is most noticeable, to begin the decluttering process. Commence the evaluation of the area visually, noting any areas that are notably disorganized or congested. This preliminary survey will assist you in establishing a strategy and prioritizing areas that require decluttering.

After determining which room requires attention, divide it into more manageable sections or categories. An illustration of this would be beginning the decluttering process in the bedroom with the closet, progressing to the bureau, bedside tables, and so forth. You can make steady progress without feeling overburdened by concentrating your attention and energy on a single area at a time by dividing the room into manageable sections.

Before proceeding with the decluttering of each section of the room, employ a methodical strategy for organizing your belongings. Assign distinct piles or containers to each of the following categories—retaining, donating, selling, or discarding—and evaluate each item according to its practicality, worth, and pertinence to one's existence. It is important to maintain awareness of the available space within one's residence and refrain from holding onto items out of obligation or remorse.

Maintain momentum during the cleansing process by establishing attainable objectives and commemorating your advancements. Every minor achievement, from organizing an entire room to clearing out a single compartment, brings you one step closer to your ultimate objective of creating a more streamlined and streamlined living space.

One can approach the task of simplifying their home one space at a time by decluttering in a systematic manner, moving from room to room. You will regain a sense of tranquility, insight, and autonomy in your living space as each area is decluttered of superfluous and unwarranted possessions.

The Minimalist Values

When striving to streamline our lives and reduce congestion, it is critical to apply the tenets of minimalism—a philosophical movement that prioritizes intentionality over impulsiveness, simplicity over excess, and quality over quantity. By adopting minimalist principles, individuals can enhance their ability to discern and decide what to retain, discard, and how to furnish a space that mirrors their personal values and priorities.

A fundamental principle of minimalism entails possessing a reduced number of items, yet ensuring that each one is of superior quality and holds significant value. This entails the meticulous curation of a collection of possessions that fulfill a functional function and elicit happiness, as opposed to the mere accumulation of items for the sake of accumulation. By prioritizing quality over quantity, one can foster a more intentional relationship with their belongings and reduce the presence of congestion.

Consistently simplifying and decluttering our living spaces constitutes an additional foundational tenet of minimalism. This entails consistently evaluating our belongings and relinquishing anything that has ceased to function or is inconsistent with our principles. Through the regular practice of decluttering our residences, we can avert the accumulation of debris and maintain living areas that are functional, well-organized, and promote a feeling of serenity and peace.

Marie Kondo, an authority on decluttering, popularized the Kon-Mari method, which draws inspiration from minimalist principles. This approach promotes the notion that individuals should evaluate their belongings according to their ability to "spark joy" and dispose of anything that fails to do so. The KonMari method promotes a more deliberate and mindful approach to decluttering through an emphasis on the emotional significance of our possessions.

There are numerous additional minimalist principles and techniques besides the KonMari method that can serve as a guide for our decluttering endeavors. There are an infinite number of methods for incorporating minimalism into our daily lives, ranging from the 333 Challenge, which requires us to reduce our inventory to 33 items, to the one-in, one-out rule, which states that for each new item introduced into the house, one must be removed.

By applying minimalist principles to the process of decluttering, one can establish a living environment that is not solely devoid of superfluous items and disorderly possessions, but also in accordance with one's personal values and priorities. Achieving greater clarity, simplicity, and fulfillment in our lives is possible through minimalism, which enables us to concentrate on what is truly essential and relinquish the remainder.

Strategies for Making Decisions

Decision-making regarding which items to retain, donate, or discard can be among the most difficult aspects of the decluttering process. Nevertheless, by implementing efficient decision-making techniques, we can facilitate this procedure and guarantee that the decluttering is carried out with intention and clarity.

A beneficial approach is to commence with the low-hanging fruit, which consists of straightforward choices that demand little exertion or reflection. Commence the process by discerning articles that are manifestly obsolete or inconsequential to one's existence, including duplicates, damaged or unused possessions, or expired products. As you progress through the decluttering process, you can attract attention and acquire confidence by beginning with these simple decisions.

Then, arrange items in order of importance, value, and practicality in relation to your daily existence. When contemplating each individual object, inquire whether it fulfills a functional purpose, elicits happiness, or contributes value to one's existence. If the response is negative, it might be appropriate to relinquish the situation. Exercise discerning judgment when making decisions, retaining exclusively those items that correspond to your personal values and priorities.

Before making any decisions regarding a particular item, weigh the potential consequences of keeping or discarding it. Would maintaining this item promote an untidy and disorderly living environment, or would it contribute to your sense of serenity and peace? You can ensure that your living space reflects your values and priorities by approaching decision-making with a greater awareness of its repercussions.

An additional effective approach to decision-making involves establishing restrictions or boundaries for particular categories of items. For instance, you might restrict the number of apparel items in your wardrobe or the quantity of books in your collection. Establishing these limits can aid in the prevention of disarray and guarantee the ability to uphold a more efficient and structured living area.

Ultimately, exercise self-compassion during the entirety of the decision-making procedure. Empathies and attachments to possessions may be evoked during the decluttering process, making it challenging to let go. Permit yourself to recognize these emotions without passing judgment, and grant yourself the authority to relinquish possessions that have ceased to be useful. Keep in mind that the process of decluttering is an ongoing one, and that it is acceptable to proceed incrementally.

You can streamline the decluttering process and produce a living space that is more congruent with your values and priorities by implementing efficient decision-making techniques. Have faith in your ability to make decisions that are in your best interests, and permit yourself to relinquish anything that no longer contributes value to your life or brings you pleasure.

Handling Sentimentimental Items

One of the most formidable components of the decluttering process entails handling sentimental items—belongings that possess deep emotional meaning and elicit cherished recollections. Emotionally distressing is the process of relinquishing sentimental objects, such as personal mementos, love letters, or family heirlooms. Nonetheless, it is possible to pay homage to these recollections while efficiently decluttering with the proper methodology.

It is essential to recognize and respect the emotions that arise as a preliminary step when decluttering sentimental belongings. Permit oneself to reflect upon the recollections linked to each object and articulate any emotions of nostalgia, sorrow, or emotional connection that emerge. By granting yourself permission to experience these feelings, you can constructively and healthily process them.

Following this, evaluate the significance of each sentimental item in your life. Is it a source of happiness and a means of strengthening your connection to the past, or does it merely consume space and contribute to the accumulation of mess? Assess the personal worth of each item and determine whether it corresponds with your present objectives and priorities.

When evaluating each sentimental item, consider whether it fulfills a practical function or elicits authentic joy. If the item enhances your existence and brings you happiness, you should absolutely retain it. However, contemplate relinquishing the item if it has ceased to fulfill a function or fail to elicit pleasure.

When deliberating on the retention or disposal of sentimental possessions, one should contemplate alternative methods of safeguarding the corresponding memories. For instance, envision digitizing a collection of sentimental letters and documents or capturing photographs of sentimental items prior to their disposal. You can effectively declutter while honouring the past by devising inventive methods of preserving memories without clinging to physical possessions.

In conclusion, maintain self-compassion and patience as you declutter sentimental belongings. When relinquishing cherished possessions, it is normal to experience a sense of melancholy or sorrow. However, bear in mind that the memories associated with these items will endure regardless of whether the physical objects are retained. By deliberately and mindfully decluttering, one can furnish a living space that is devoid of excess while simultaneously imbued with significance and happiness.

4

Chapter 4: Simplifying Your Digital Life

Digital Repository

Our lives are becoming more and more intertwined with technology in the current digital age, which has led to a proliferation of digital detritus that can be overwhelming and impede productivity. In order to establish a more streamlined and efficient digital environment and reclaim authority over our digital lives, it is imperative to commence by performing an exhaustive digital inventory.

Conduct an inventory of your digital assets encompassing files, emails, photographs, and applications, which are dispersed across multiple devices and platforms. By conducting this thorough inventory, you will gain a precise understanding of the magnitude of your digital detritus and be able to pinpoint specific areas that require decluttering and organization.

Pay close attention to duplicates, obsolete files, and irrelevant content that may be clogging your digital space as you conduct your digital inventory. Leverage software and tools to aid in the identification and classification of digital detritus, thereby facilitating the prioritization of areas requiring decluttering and optimization.

Systematically arrange your digital inventory by establishing folders and subfolders for the purpose of classifying files and documents in a manner that is both logical and intuitive. Implement standardized naming conventions and file organization systems in order to streamline the process of retrieving and managing digital assets.

Do not overlook evaluating your digital communication channels, such as messaging applications, social media accounts, and files and documents. To reduce digital noise and distractions, unsubscribe from superfluous email subscriptions, declutter your inbox by archiving or deleting old emails, and streamline your social media feeds.

By performing an exhaustive digital inventory and proficiently organizing your digital assets, you will establish the groundwork for a digital environment that is more streamlined and fruitful. Not only will regaining authority over your digital inundation result in time and frustration savings, but it will also create cognitive capacity for more significant endeavors and life experiences.

Methods of Organization

After undertaking an exhaustive digital inventory, the subsequent course of action entails executing organizational strategies that aim to optimize one's digital existence. One can increase productivity, decrease tension, and establish a more streamlined digital workflow by effectively organizing digital files, documents, and communication channels.

To commence, organize and streamline your digital files and documents by implementing the tenets of minimalism into your digital environment. Methodically examine the contents of your files, eliminating duplicates, obsolete documents, and superfluous files that have lost their functionality. In order to facilitate simple retrieval, arrange the remaining files into folders and subfolders, grouping similar items together and employing descriptive file names.

One should contemplate the implementation of a cloud-based storage solution as a means to consolidate and synchronize digital files across an assortment of devices. Cloud storage services provide users with the ability to seamlessly collaborate with others and access their files from any location, while also providing convenience, accessibility, and scalability. To protect your digital assets, select a reputable cloud storage provider that places a high emphasis on data privacy and security.

Enhance productivity and efficiency by optimizing digital workflows in addition to file organization. Determine which aspects of your digital routine are repetitive and investigate software and automation tools that can be utilized to streamline them. By utilizing productivity applications and tools, one can efficiently monitor deadlines, prioritize projects, and manage tasks, thereby reducing feelings of being overwhelmed and increasing overall productivity.

Optimize your digital communication channels in order to reduce interruptions and improve concentration. Organize your email inboxes by consolidating them, deactivating unused subscriptions, and establishing labels and filters to prioritize critical messages. By centralizing and streamlining team collaboration with the aid of communication apps and tools, the necessity for back-and-forth correspondence and meetings is diminished.

Your digital environment will be more harmonious and fruitful as a result of the organizational strategies you employ to streamline your digital life. In today's digital world, regaining control of your digital detritus and optimizing your digital workflows will not only increase your productivity and efficiency, but also your well-being and quality of life.

Electronic Detox

In a time characterized by the pervasiveness of digital devices and online connectivity, the burden of constant notifications, information inundation, and the expectation to remain constantly connected can be tremendous. A digital detox provides an opportunity to disconnect from the constant onslaught of digital stimuli, enabling individuals to reacquaint themselves with their surroundings and reestablish connection with their devices.

To begin, establish limits on your digital usage by designating specific times and locations for activities that do not involve the use of digital devices. Establish designated periods of the day, such as before bed or during mealtimes, as sacred no-screen zones. During these periods, concentrate on being fully present and engaged with oneself, one's loved ones, or one's surroundings.

It is advisable to contemplate the adoption of digital-free days or weekends, during which one abstains from using digital devices and platforms in favor of offline pursuits that provide mental, physical, and spiritual nourishment. During this period, devote yourself to personal interests, immerse yourself in natural surroundings, or establish meaningful connections with loved ones in person, unencumbered by electronic devices and notifications.

Make it a priority to engage in activities that foster self-care, relaxation, and mindfulness throughout your digital detox. Engage in deep breathing exercises, yoga, or meditation to cultivate inner calm and quiet the mind. Indulge in pursuits that elicit feelings of joy and satisfaction, such as strolling through a park, engaging in artistic endeavors, or perusing scholarly works.

Establish a conducive atmosphere for your digital detox by enlisting the assistance of family, friends, or accountability companions. Promote your resolution to abstain from digital devices and solicit the support of others in adopting a similar digital detox regimen. As you navigate the difficulties and benefits of disconnecting, hold one another accountable and offer encouragement and support.

Engaging in a digital detox will result in an enhanced state of equilibrium, concentration, and clarity in one's life. By disengaging from digital devices, one can reclaim their time and attention, thereby nurturing more profound connections with both themselves and others, as well as developing a heightened sense of presence and mindfulness in every moment.

Optimising Devices and Applications

App overflow is a prevalent issue in the contemporary digital environment, wherein smartphones and tablets are overloaded with an abundance of applications competing for our focus. It is crucial to optimize your applications and devices in order to simplify your digital existence and enhance the user experience by promoting concentration and efficiency.

Beginning with an audit of your devices and applications, determine which ones are indispensable to your daily activities and duties. One should contemplate the removal or deactivation of applications that are seldom utilized or perform redundant functions, in order to liberate valuable storage space and diminish digital detritus.

When it comes to applications, prioritize quality over quantity, concentrating on those that provide the greatest functionality and value. Select applications that are intuitive, dependable, and in accordance with your particular requirements and inclinations. Exercise discernment when choosing applications; refrain from downloading each novel app that claims to bring about a significant transformation in your life.

Devices should be organized with folders or categories containing applications in order to reduce congestion and facilitate access. Classify applications with comparable functions or purposes, such as fitness apps, entertainment apps, or productivity apps. Develop an optimized application layout that aligns with your digital objectives and improves usability.

One should contemplate embracing a minimalist aesthetic when it comes to their digital devices, prioritizing functionality and simplicity over extraneous features and functions. Opt for devices that fulfill your particular requirements while avoiding superfluous functions or intricacy. It is advisable to maintain streamlined and uncluttered device settings, preventing excessive notifications and cluttered home displays.

Review and update your devices and applications on a regular basis to ensure they continue to satisfy your requirements and preferences. It is advisable to remove obsolete or unused applications from your device and conduct regular evaluations of its settings and configurations in order to enhance performance and efficiency. You will generate a more concentrated and streamlined digital experience that increases productivity and decreases digital overload by streamlining your applications and devices.

Privacy and Security of Data

As the world becomes more interconnected, data security and privacy concerns have assumed paramount importance. In the current digital era, protecting your personal information and digital assets is crucial for defending against cyber threats and ensuring your peace of mind.

Commence by acquiring knowledge regarding prevalent cybersecurity threats and optimal methodologies for safeguarding one's data. Maintain awareness of the most recent security breaches and vulnerabilities, and fortify your devices and accounts against potential threats by taking preventative measures. To maintain the security of your devices and accounts, implement robust passwords, enable two-factor authentication, and update your software and security settings on a regular basis.

It is imperative to exercise caution when disclosing information online and on social media platforms, as cybercriminals may exploit vulnerabilities and single you out for identity theft or fraud using even apparently innocuous details. Review and exercise caution when disclosing personal information, and manage your privacy settings to determine who has access to it and how it is utilized.

Maintaining regular backups of your digital data safeguards against data loss caused by hardware failure, larceny, or other unforeseen circumstances. Implement redundancy measures by utilizing external hard drives or cloud-based backup services to duplicate critical files and documents. This will guarantee their retrieval in the event of a catastrophic event or data breach.

One should contemplate making an investment in cybersecurity software and services as a means to fortify their digital security stance. Virtual private networks (VPNs), antivirus software, and firewalls can assist in safeguarding your devices and data against phishing attacks, malware, and other cyber threats. Select cybersecurity providers of high repute who place a high priority on data security and privacy in order to effectively protect your digital assets.

By placing a high value on data security and privacy in your online activities, you will reduce the likelihood of encountering cyber threats and safeguard your personal information against unauthorized access or improper use. Implementing preventive security measures for your devices, accounts, and data will provide you with reassurance and enable you to confidently and securely navigate the digital realm.

5

❧

Chapter 5: Minimalist Living Spaces

Design Fundamentals

The creation of minimalist living spaces is influenced by core design principles that place an emphasis on functionality, intentionality, and simplicity. The foundation of minimalist design is the notion of simplicity—a dedication to reducing superfluous elements and emphasizing the critical components that foster a cohesive habitation space.

Minimalist design is characterized by uncluttered spaces, pure lines, and a restrained color scheme. By removing superfluous embellishments and decorative components, minimalist living spaces foster an atmosphere of serenity and peace, which is conducive to relaxation and overall health.

An additional tenet of minimalist design is functionality, which emphasizes the significance of areas that facilitate the daily activities and procedures of the occupants and serve a practical purpose.

Each component within a minimalist living environment is deliberately chosen based on its practicality and impact on the overall functionality of the room.

The foundation of minimalist design is intentionality, which influences each decision and selection that is undertaken during the development of a living environment. Every component of a minimalist living environment is deliberately and conscientiously selected, ranging from furnishings and decorations to the arrangement and structure of the room.

The process of amending and refining these design principles into one's personal living space is intentional when attempting to incorporate them. Commence the process by decluttering and streamlining your environment by eliminating any objects that lack functionality or fail to elicit happiness. By embracing open spaces and clear, uncluttered lines, you enable every element in your home to flourish and illuminate.

You can create a minimalist living space that embodies your values and priorities, promotes serenity and calmness, and facilitates your transition to a more uncomplicated and purposeful lifestyle by adhering to the design principles of functionality, intentionality, and simplicity.

De-cluttering Methods

The implementation of efficient decluttering methods is critical in order to convert living areas into tranquil havens characterized by simplicity and minimalism. By employing these strategies, people are able to methodically streamline every space in their residences, resulting in more airy and structured settings that foster tranquility and health.

Initiate the process of decluttering by decomposing each room in your residence into feasible assignments. Begin by addressing high-traffic areas such as the kitchen, living room, or entryway, and then systematically progress to the remaining areas of the residence.

Without feeling overburdened, one can sustain focus and momentum by addressing each area individually.

Implement a methodical strategy when arranging your possessions as you declutter each space. In order to determine which items to retain, donate, sell, or discard, partition them into distinct piles or containers according to their practicality, worth, and pertinence to one's existence. Demonstrate ruthlessness in your decision-making process, relinquishing anything that has ceased to be functional or enjoyable.

One should contemplate the adoption of the KonMari approach, formulated by the renowned decluttering expert Marie Kondo. This approach advocates for the evaluation of one's possessions according to their ability to evoke pleasure. This method encourages a more deliberate and conscious approach to the process of decluttering, with the goal of retaining exclusively those items that evoke a profound emotional response and enhance one's overall state of contentment and well-being.

An additional efficacious method for decluttering is adhering to the one-in, one-out rule: for each additional item introduced into the household, one must be eliminated. This regulation serves to inhibit the gradual accumulation of detritus and promotes a more deliberate stance towards acquisition and consumption.

Through the implementation of these decluttering strategies, one can effectively convert their living areas into minimalist havens devoid of superfluous items and disarray. With perseverance and fortitude, embrace the process, recognizing that every stage brings you one step closer to establishing a residence that fosters and sustains your overall welfare.

Multipurpose Furnishings

The deliberate choice of furniture is crucial in the pursuit of minimalist living as it enables the most efficient use of available space and functionality. Multifunctional furniture has emerged as a pivotal solution, providing exceptional comfort and design while simultaneously ensuring versatility and efficiency.

By selecting pieces that serve multiple purposes, one can optimize the practicality of their living area, especially in smaller or more congested settings. It is advisable to contemplate making an investment in multifunctional furniture, such as a coffee table featuring storage compartments or a sofa bed. These multipurpose pieces not only optimize living space but also augment the practicality of one's residence by accommodating a range of requirements and activities.

An additional benefit of multifunctional furniture is its capacity to foster adaptability and flexibility in the living area. By utilizing furniture that is readily transformable or reconfigurable, one can customize their environment to suit various activities or occasions such as working remotely, entertaining guests, or unwinding in solitude. This adaptability permits your living space to develop in tandem with you, to accommodate your shifting preferences and requirements.

Furniture that serves multiple purposes can enhance the visual attractiveness of a space, in addition to their practical utility. Numerous contemporary designs effectively harmonize aesthetics and practicality, presenting streamlined and fashionable resolutions that augment the overall ambiance of one's living area. By selecting multifunctional furniture that reflects your personal style and preferences, it is possible to create a visually appealing and functional minimalist environment.

Prioritize craftsmanship and quality when integrating multifunctional furniture into your home in order to guarantee its longevity and durability. Opt for durable, well-designed pieces constructed with materials and attention to detail that can withstand the test of time. Purchasing high-quality furniture not only improves the operational capacity of a given area but also contributes to the long-term value of a residence.

A minimalist living space can be optimized in terms of space, functionality, and aesthetics through the incorporation of multi-functional furniture. By employing strategic selection and deliberate design principles, multifunctional pieces have the capacity to revolutionize one's living space into a flexible and adaptable sanctuary that mirrors one's personal values of efficiency and simplicity.

Relocation Solutions

Efficient storage solutions are critical for the maintenance of a minimalist living space that is devoid of debris and well-organized. By optimizing storage capacity and reducing visual disorderliness, one can establish an environment conducive to tranquility and serenity.

Commence the process by conducting a storage requirements assessment and categorizing areas that necessitate supplementary storage solutions. To optimize storage capacity without invading valuable floor space, contemplate making use of underutilized areas such as walls, corners, and vertical surfaces. To maintain an orderly and uncluttered appearance while keeping frequently used items easily accessible, consider installing shelves, pegs, and organizers.

Consider incorporating built-in storage options into your home's architecture to optimize space utilization and incorporate storage solutions seamlessly. Designed to accommodate individual preferences and requirements, built-in shelving, drawers, and cabinets offer discrete storage solutions that complement a minimalist aesthetic.

To maximise space utilisation and minimise visual congestion, consider investing in multifunctional furniture that incorporates storage compartments in its design. To optimize storage space while upholding a streamlined and unified aesthetic, consider purchasing coffee tables with lift-top surfaces, ottomans featuring concealed compartments, and mattresses equipped with storage drawers.

Adopt minimalist storage containers and organizers in order to maintain readily accessible and well-organized belongings. Select receptacles and organizers featuring sleek and uncomplicated designs that harmonize with your minimalist décor and amplify the overall visual appeal of your living area.

It is imperative to consistently engage in decluttering and purging of superfluous items in order to avert storage spaces from becoming inundated with an excess of possessions. Embrace a mindset characterized by deliberate acquisition and intentional consumption, placing a premium on quality rather than quantity, and allocate your resources towards products that enhance your life in terms of utility and worth.

You can create a functional and aesthetically appealing minimalist living space through the implementation of efficient storage solutions. By applying strategic storage solutions and meticulous organization, one can effectively manage household debris, thereby fostering an atmosphere conducive to relaxation, productivity, and overall well-being.

Deliberate Décor

Within the domain of minimalist living, each ornamental component fulfills a specific function, thereby augmenting the ambiance and aesthetic appeal of the entire space. A tranquil and harmonious atmosphere that mirrors one's individuality and values is largely attributable to the conscientious selection of décor.

Commence the process by curating a compilation of decorative objects that adhere to the tenets of minimalism, namely intentionality, functionality, and simplicity. Select decorative items that emanate a feeling of serenity and peace; favor natural materials, neutral hues, and sleek silhouettes that harmonize with your minimalist design philosophy.

When choosing decor items, place an emphasis on quality rather than quantity. Invest in exquisitely crafted pieces that will endure the passage of time and add delight to your living space. Select decorative and functional items for the space, such as a sculptural vase or a stylish timepiece, which not only add aesthetic appeal but also fulfill a practical function.

By utilizing negative space as a design element, you can create an atmosphere in your home that is devoid of embellishment and disorder. By incorporating vacant space into your design scheme in a strategic manner, you enhance the overall flow and vitality of the room by establishing a sense of equilibrium and transparency.

Choose decorative elements with intention, specifically those that possess personal significance or meaning to you. Incorporate personal mementos, cherished photographs, artwork, and hand-crafted treasures that elicit positive emotions and bring pleasure into your living space.

Consistently reevaluate your selection of décor and simplify your collection as necessary in order to preserve an aesthetically pleasing and uncluttered setting. By adopting the principle of "less is more," eliminate any decorative elements that have outlived their usefulness or fail to correspond with your personal aesthetic preferences.

One can cultivate a minimalist living space that is profoundly significant and aesthetically pleasing by adopting a mindful and purposeful approach to decor. Every individual decorative element enhances the ambiance and vitality of the room, promoting a feeling of tranquility, equilibrium, and health within your residence.

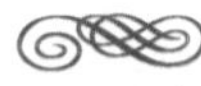

Chapter 6: Cultivating Minimalist Habits

Constant Routines

The foundation of developing a more refined and purposeful lifestyle lies in the incorporation of minimalist principles into one's daily routines. One can lay the groundwork for a more harmonious and gratifying existence by integrating simplicity and mindfulness into every facet of their daily routine.

To commence, conduct an analysis of your existing daily regimens to pinpoint potential areas for the integration of parsimonious practices. Commence with your morning routine, establishing the ambiance for the forthcoming day through deliberate actions that foster lucidity and concentration. By removing superfluous steps and diversions from your morning routine, you can enable yourself to commence the day with a sense of tranquility and intention.

Engage in mindful practices throughout the day, incorporating awareness into every instant of your interactions and activities, and embracing the aesthetic value of simplicity. Engage in activities that promote mindfulness, such as sipping tea in silence, strolling through natural surroundings, or pursuing creative endeavors. Attempt to find moments to decelerate and completely appreciate the present moment.

Unwind at the end of the day by employing a minimalist strategy for self-care and relaxation. Establish a soothing twilight routine that facilitates a state of sound sleep and adequately equips you for the upcoming day. Discharge from electronic devices, lower the illumination, and partake in activities that foster tranquility and relaxation, such as engaging in mild yoga, reading, or journaling.

By integrating minimalist principles into one's daily routines, an atmosphere of cadence and fluidity can be established, which serves to elevate one's overall state of being. By streamlining your daily routines, you are able to concentrate on what is truly significant, fostering a more profound sense of self-awareness and connection with the world. Developing the practice of mindful and intentional presence in every moment will transform your daily routines into sources of happiness, satisfaction, and significance.

Conscious Consumption

Promoting a more deliberate and environmentally conscious way of life through conscientious consumption is essential to the pursuit of minimalism. Through the implementation of conscious consumerism principles, individuals can enhance their ability to select experiences over material possessions, thereby prioritizing experiences over waste reduction and material possessions.

Commence your purchasing endeavors by establishing unambiguous standards, prioritizing longevity, functionality, and quality over quantity or fashion. Deliberate on the environmental and personal ramifications of every purchase, selecting items that are consistent with your personal values and fulfill an authentic function.

Adopt the principle of "one in, one out" as a governing framework to ensure that your living space is devoid of clutter. Make a personal pledge to relinquish an existing item for each additional item you acquire, encompassing household products, apparel, and electronic devices. Engaging in this activity not only inhibits the accumulation of debris but also promotes conscientious consumption and purposeful living.

Replace an emphasis on material possessions with an emphasis on experiences and interpersonal connections. Invest in experiences that bring you joy and fulfillment, such as traveling, developing a hobby, or spending precious time with loved ones, as opposed to amassing more material possessions. Develop significant relationships and recollections that enhance one's life considerably more than material gains could.

Develop an attitude of appreciation for the abundance that is already a part of your life; instead of perpetually seeking more, cultivate gratitude for what you possess. Develop an intrinsic sense of satisfaction and contentment, as opposed to pursuing validation or fulfillment from the outside through material possessions.

Through mindful consumption, one can foster a more profound sense of satisfaction, connection, and meaning in one's existence. We can establish a more meaningful and sustainable way of life that is consistent with our values and improves the prospects for both ourselves and the planet through deliberate decision-making regarding our consumption and lifestyle.

Minimalism in Digital

Cultivating minimalist practices in the digital age means expanding its reach beyond physical possessions to encompass one's digital life. Intentionally simplifying our relationship with technology in order to reduce feelings of being overwhelmed, reclaim time and attention, and cultivate greater clarity and presence in our lives is the goal of digital minimalism.

Establish limits on your digital usage by designating specific times and locations for technological purposes. Create designated areas without electronic devices in your residence, such as the dining room or bedroom, where you can engage in offline activities and interactions without the presence of screens.

Declutter your digital devices, such as smartphones, tablets, and computers, on a regular basis in order to eliminate digital clutter and distractions. Minimize digital overload and enhance cognitive clarity by optimizing notification systems, removing unused applications, and organizing files and folders.

Engage in periodic digital detoxes in order to recharge and restore your relationship with technology. Designate specific time intervals, such as vacations or weekends, during which you refrain from using digital devices and engage in offline pursuits that provide nourishment for your physical, mental, and spiritual well-being.

By establishing limits on one's screen time, engaging in digital mindfulness exercises, and prioritizing significant connections over aimless perusing, one can cultivate mindful technological practices. By deliberately employing technology to augment your life rather than divert attention from it, prioritize activities that are consistent with your personal values and objectives.

Adopt digital applications and tools that facilitate a minimalist way of life, including productivity and meditation applications, as well as digital decluttering tools. Opt for technological devices that optimize efficiency and productivity, while reducing interruptions and feelings of being overwhelmed.

By reclaiming our time and attention for what truly matters in life, we can establish a more balanced and purposeful relationship with technology through the application of digital minimalism. Develop a heightened sense of presence, connection, and fulfillment in the contemporary digital era by adopting digital practices that prioritize mindfulness and simplicity.

Ecological Sustainability

Minimalist practices promote environmental sustainability by incentivizing individuals to reduce pollution, consume fewer items, and live more sustainably on the planet. We can minimize our ecological imprint and contribute to a more sustainable and health-conscious future for ourselves and future generations by adopting minimalist practices.

Beginning with a less-is-more mentality, decrease your over-all consumption. When making purchases, prioritize quality over quantity by selecting durable and long-lasting products that reduce the frequency of replacements. By purchasing products manufactured in an environmentally responsible manner and using sustainable materials, you are endorsing businesses that place a premium on ethical and eco-friendly operations.

Reduce waste by implementing strategies such as decomposition, recycling, and the reduction of single-use plastics. When making purchases, exercise caution regarding packaging by selecting items with minimal packaging or packaging that can be recycled or biodegradated. To lower your environmental footprint and reduce waste, contemplate reusable alternatives to disposable items, including water bottles, purchasing bags, and food containers.

Adopt a minimalist transportation philosophy by decreasing dependence on fossil fuels and, whenever feasible, utilizing public transportation, walking, bicycling, or cycling. Carpooling and ridesharing are viable alternatives that can be utilized to mitigate the environmental consequences of travel by reducing emissions.

By investing in energy-efficient appliances and lighting, turning off lights and electronics when not in use, and utilizing programmable thermostats to control heating and cooling, you can reduce your home's energy consumption. When feasible, incorporate natural ventilation and light to minimize reliance on artificial illumination and air conditioning.

Foster environmental preservation initiatives and advocate for policies that safeguard the planet and advance sustainability. Participate in community initiatives, volunteer with environmental organizations, and advocate for positive change by using your voice to bring attention to environmental issues.

By incorporating environmentally sustainable practices and imbibing minimalist habits, we can mitigate our ecological impact and make a positive contribution towards a more resilient and sustainable planet. Every minor adjustment we implement on a daily basis possesses the capacity to impact positively and establish a more promising future for both present and future generations.

Engaging in Mindfulness Practices

It is crucial to incorporate mindfulness practices into our daily lives in order to foster a heightened state of presence, consciousness, and interior tranquility in the face of the hectic pace of contemporary existence. By cultivating an attitude of inquiry and attentiveness towards the present moment, mindfulness facilitates a more profound connection with oneself, others, and the environment.

Commence by integrating mindfulness practices into your daily regimen, such as yoga, meditation, or deep breathing exercises. Whether it be a brief moment of mindful breathing before bed, a session of meditation in the morning, or a yoga session during your lunch break, set aside time each day to engage in these practices. Through the deliberate allocation of time for the practice of mindfulness, one can develop an enhanced state of tranquility and equilibrium that permeates every facet of existence.

Engage in daily activities with mindfulness, directing one's attention and consciousness towards the present moment as it transpires. Engage in activities such as conversing, strolling through nature, and consuming food with your entire being present. Do so by attentively observing your thoughts, feelings, and sensations without passing judgment. You can increase your sense of happiness, appreciation, and satisfaction in life by developing mindfulness in the midst of your daily activities.

Employ mindfulness practices to facilitate stress management and enhance one's mental health. Pinch and recall to the present moment while taking a few deep breaths during times of tension or overwhelm. Employ mindfulness techniques, such as progressive muscle relaxation or body assessments, to alleviate stress and foster mental and physical relaxation.

Promote mindfulness in interpersonal connections through the application of compassionate and empathetic listening. Listen with an open mind and heart while interacting with others, maintaining complete presence and focus. Develop comprehension and empathy by placing oneself in the shoes of another and considering the situation from their vantage point. Through the practice of mindfulness, one can nurture more profound and gratifying connections within their personal life.

An increased state of awareness, well-being, and presence can be developed through the daily incorporation of mindfulness practices. Observe as mindfulness imparts inner-soul transformation, fostering greater serenity, joy, and fulfillment in every aspect of your life, as you approach each moment with curiosity and receptivity.

7

Chapter 7: Minimalism Beyond Material Possessions

Acceptance of Inner Minimalism

Although the concept of minimalist living frequently centers around the reduction of material possessions, authentic minimalism transcends this and encompasses the internal environment as well. By encouraging us to simplify our souls and minds, inner minimalism promotes mental clarity, emotional health, and spiritual development.

Before adopting inner minimalism, purge your mind of all unnecessary items. Similar to how we declutter our living spaces, we can liberate our minds from congestion by relinquishing unproductive negative thoughts, concerns, and constraining convictions. By cultivating mindfulness, one can impartially observe and acknowledge one's thoughts, permitting them to transiently dissipate like clouds in the sky.

Embrace emotional simplicity through the development of sound boundaries and the release of exhausting obligations and toxic relationships. Create a circle of individuals who inspire and uplift you, thereby cultivating more profound relationships founded on sincerity, reliance, and reciprocal regard. The act of simplifying relationships enables individuals to allocate their time and effort towards cultivating significant connections that enhance the quality of life.

Spiritual minimalism promotes the practice of eliminating extraneous elements and establishing a connection with one's innermost being. Establish periods of silence and stillness, whether by means of prayer, meditation, or other contemplative practices, in order to commune with your intuition and interior wisdom. By streamlining our spiritual practices, we can attain a more profound union with the divine and manifest increased tranquility and satisfaction in our existence.

The pursuit of interior minimalism necessitates a continuous process of introspection and self-realization. We create an environment conducive to the growth of clarity, creativity, and inspiration by simplifying our thoughts and emotions. By relinquishing material possessions that have ceased to benefit us and reestablishing harmony with our fundamental nature, we initiate the profound influence of interior minimalism, which enables us to lead lives imbued with more meaning, awareness, and happiness.

Simplifying Interpersonal Relations

Within the domain of minimalist living, the imperative of simplifying relationships is frequently disregarded despite its critical nature. Similar to how we streamline our living spaces and improve visibility by removing unnecessary items, simplifying interpersonal connections enables us to cultivate more profound bonds, establish limits, and give precedence to significant connections that are consistent with our values and bring us happiness.

Determine which relationships in your life energize and elevate you, as opposed to those that deplete and exhaust you, by conducting an assessment of your personal relationships. Assess the degree of mutual respect and support, the quality of your interactions, and the congruence between the relationship and your personal values and objectives. Abandon relationships that have ceased to contribute to your development or welfare, thereby liberating yourself from the weight of detrimental dynamics or unidirectional connections.

Protect your time, energy, and emotional well-being in relationships by establishing healthy boundaries. Clearly and assertively communicate your expectations and requirements, establishing boundaries regarding your willingness and capability to receive and contribute. Placing self-care and self-respect as top priorities entails declining obligations or requests that are incongruent with one's values or priorities.

Develop more profound relationships with individuals who hold the utmost importance in your life by devoting time and effort to fostering substantial connections founded on sincerity, reliance, and reciprocal regard. Place an emphasis on quality rather than quantity, giving depth and intimacy precedence over superficiality and quantity. Construct a network of individuals who are supportive in nature and who inspire and motivate you, reflecting your values and ambitions.

Employ empathy and compassion in your interpersonal interactions, making an effort to comprehend the viewpoints and experiences of others with a receptive and unbiased attitude. Actively and attentively listen, validate the emotions and experiences of others, and provide encouragement and support when necessary. By cultivating empathy and understanding, one can nurture a sense of connection and belonging in interpersonal relationships, as well as strengthen existing bonds.

A continuous process of self-discovery and development, relationship simplification requires introspection, fortitude, and dedication. By establishing boundaries, decluttering toxic relationships, and fostering meaningful connections, one can make room in their life for genuine and satisfying connections that enhance their well-being and enrich the individual experience.

Effective Time Management

Minimalist time management entails the establishment of boundaries, the prioritization of tasks, and the acceptance of the ability to decline commitments that fail to correspond with our objectives and priorities. Amidst an ever-expanding array of obligations and diversions, attaining proficiency in parsimonious time management strategies can enable us to reclaim authority over our timetables and concentrate on matters that genuinely require our attention.

Commence by identifying your short-term and long-term objectives and priorities. Which pursuits and activities bestow upon you feelings of delight, satisfaction, and a sense of direction? You can allocate your time and energy more efficiently by establishing clear priorities, concentrating on endeavors that are in line with your values and advance you toward your objectives.

Create clear parameters for your time and effort in order to mitigate the risk of exhaustion and mental burden. Develop the ability to decline commitments and requests that are incongruent with one's personal values and priorities. This will liberate oneself from superfluous responsibilities and allow one to allocate more energy to matters that truly matter. Clearly delineate limits regarding working hours, personal time, and self-care, placing daily emphasis on equilibrium and wellness.

Adopt minimalist approaches to time management, such as time blocking, which entails designating distinct time intervals for various activities and duties. By allocating uninterrupted, focused time to each task, one can optimize productivity and efficiency while reducing interruptions and the need to multitask. Prioritize tasks according to their urgency and significance, addressing the most important duties initially and delegating or delaying the less important ones as necessary.

Adopting a mindfulness-based time management strategy entails maintaining attention on the current task while avoiding distractions and feelings of being overwhelmed. By employing mindfulness techniques, such as deep breathing or grounding exercises, one can achieve inner peace and maintain mental lucidity in the midst of the fast-paced nature of daily existence.

Achieving proficiency in minimalist time management techniques can lead to the development of a more harmonious, meaningful, and satisfying existence. You can empower yourself to live with intention and purpose in today's fast-paced world by cultivating greater focus, productivity, and well-being through the alignment of your time and energy with your priorities and values.

Cognitive Clutter

It is essential, in the pursuit of minimalist living, to address the mental clutter that exists in addition to the clutter that fills our physical environments. Mental clutter occurs when our mental space becomes inundated with an onslaught of concerns, worries, and diversions. This can impede our capacity to concentrate, reach resolutions, and attain interior tranquility.

Prior to decluttering our thoughts, we must identify the origins of mental clutter in our daily activities. This may manifest as persistent preoccupation with future events, mental reenactment of past occurrences, or fixation on negative thoughts and emotions. We can begin to resolve these patterns and create an environment conducive to tranquility and clarity by recognizing them.

Mindfulness meditation is a potent instrument for mental

purification. By engaging in consistent meditation, individuals develop the ability to impartially observe their thoughts, permitting them to enter and exit without becoming entangled in them. Through the practice of developing mindfulness, it is possible to still the perpetual babble of the mind and attain enhanced levels of clarity and tranquility.

Another effective method for decluttering the psyche is keeping a journal. Engaging in written expression of our thoughts and emotions can facilitate the release of mental strain and provide valuable insight into our interior selves. We are able to examine our thoughts and emotions in a secure and nonjudgmental environment through the use of journals, which aids in the processing of difficult feelings and provides perspective on our experiences.

Additionally, cognitive-behavioral techniques can assist in mental decluttering through the substitution of pessimistic thought patterns for more optimistic and empowering ones. By recognizing and reorienting erroneous thought patterns, it is possible to develop a more positive and resilient frame of mind that is beneficial to our well-being as a whole.

To provide your mind with a respite from the incessant influx of stimuli, integrate phases of silence and serenity into your daily regimen. Allowing yourself moments of serenity and quiet, whether through meditation, spending time in nature, or simply sipping tea in solitude, will help you recharge and reset.

We make room in our minds for the growth and development of lucidity, creativity, and insight by decluttering them. By incorporating mindfulness practices, journaling, and cognitive-behavioral strategies into our daily lives, we can attain enhanced tranquility, concentration, and overall welfare by clearing our minds of mental congestion.

The Search for Meaning and Purpose

The concept of minimalism transcends material possessions and encompasses an individual's profound sense of purpose and life's meaning. We can discover what truly matters to us and ensure that our actions and decisions are in line with our values and passions by adopting minimalist principles.

Consider initially what offers you happiness, satisfaction, and a sense of purpose in life. Delight in your personal values, interests, and aspirations as you discern activities and endeavors that profoundly resonate with you. You can direct your time and effort toward endeavors that gratify you and enhance your general state of being by establishing a clear sense of purpose.

Streamline your existence by eliminating obligations and diversions that are incongruent with your purpose or personal values. Detach oneself from endeavors, obligations, and material possessions that have ceased to contribute to one's development or well-being, thereby enabling the pursuit of that which is genuinely significant. Adopting a minimalist way of life where quality is prioritized over quantity, connections are valued over consumption, and experiences are favored over possessions.

Develop an attitude of gratitude towards the current abundance in your life by acknowledging and valuing the ordinary pleasures and benefits that grace your surroundings on a daily basis. Developing an attitude of gratitude enables one to redirect attention from personal shortcomings to possessions, thereby nurturing an elevated sense of satisfaction and contentment in one's existence.

Engage in activities that promote personal development and exploration, such as acquiring novel interests, expanding one's skill set, or venturing beyond one's comfort zone. Adopt challenges as prospects for personal development and expansion, placing confidence in one's capacity to surmount impediments and accomplish objectives.

You can create a life filled with significance, fulfillment, and purpose by adopting minimalist principles and remaining true to your values and intentions. You can experience greater happiness, inner serenity, and harmony by simplifying your life and concentrating on what truly matters; in doing so, you will be living in accordance with your genuine self and making a positive contribution towards a more sustainable and harmonious global community.

8

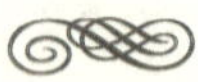

Chapter 8: Overcoming Challenges and Embracing Growth

Detecting Obstacles

Commencing a minimalistic journey is not devoid of challenges. It is imperative to recognize and comprehend the frequent challenges that may manifest throughout the process. These obstacles may include societal pressures, emotional attachments to material possessions, and resistance to change. Through the process of acknowledging and classifying these obstacles, we can enhance our readiness to confront them with fortitude and resolve.

A pervasive obstacle that frequently arises is societal pressure, which propagates materialism and consumerism as indicators of achievement and contentment. In order to defy societal norms and forge our own way, it is imperative that we must muster the fortitude and resolve to place our personal values and welfare above the approval of others.

Additionally, emotional attachment to material possessions can be a formidable obstacle on the path to minimalism. We may be compelled to cling to objects out of dread of abandonment or sentimental attachment. The process of detaching one's sense of self-worth and identity from material possessions necessitates introspection and self-reflection.

Fear of change is an additional prevalent obstacle that may impede our complete adoption of minimalism. It can be intimidating to leave our comfort zones and question the status quo, but doing so is frequently essential for personal development and change. Recognizing and confronting our anxieties enables us to proceed with bravery and resolve, recognizing that transformation is a fundamental component of the process.

By recognizing these obstacles and comprehending their fundamental origins, we can formulate tactics to surmount them and proceed with our pursuit of minimalism. By exercising patience, perseverance, and an openness to directly facing challenges, one can successfully navigate the complexities of minimalism and ultimately emerge more robust and resilient.

Developing Resilience

When striving to adopt a minimalist way of life, resilience proves to be an indispensable asset. It is the attribute that enables individuals to recover from setbacks, surmount challenges, and persevere despite the arduousness of the journey. The process of fostering resilience entails the development of fortitude, adaptive coping mechanisms, and a resilient mindset in order to effectively navigate the unavoidable obstacles that may arise.

Nurturing a growth mindset is an indispensable component of resilience. With a growth mindset, setbacks are perceived not as irreversible failings but as chances for learning and development.

Through the process of reframing obstacles as instructive experiences in fortitude and persistence, one can confront adversity with an aura of optimism and resolve.

Additionally, self-compassion is a vital component of resilience. This practice entails practicing self-compassion and empathy, particularly when confronted with adversity. Self-compassion, as opposed to negative self-criticism, enables individuals to recognize and embrace their own difficult places, thereby promoting improved emotional resilience and overall well-being.

Seeking assistance from others during the pursuit of minimalism can also enhance one's resilience. A supportive community, whether comprised of family, friends, or acquaintances, can offer invaluable perspective and encouragement by understanding and validating our experiences. By soliciting assistance when necessary, we can harness the collective intelligence and fortitude of those in our vicinity.

Engaging in self-care is a critical component of sustaining resilience and overall wellness amidst adversity. Participating in holistic practices that promote well-being, including physical activity, spiritual contemplation, and time spent immersed in nature, enables us to restore our energy levels and develop fortitude in the face of challenges and hardship.

By fostering resilience, one can confront the difficulties associated with minimalism with enhanced self-assurance, bravery, and elegance. By adopting a resilient mindset, utilizing adaptive coping mechanisms, and having a network of allies who provide support, it is possible to surmount challenges and emerge from them with increased strength, wisdom, and resilience.

Acceptance of Change

Acceptance of shifts is a fundamental component of the minimalist way of life. In the pursuit of simplifying our lives and relinquishing extravagance, we will inevitably experience periods of unpredictability, unease, and metamorphosis. Embracing change rather than resisting it enables the development of an attitude characterized by receptiveness, flexibility, and progress.

The practice of minimalism inherently entails change, as it compels us to reevaluate our priorities, values, and routines in order to conform to our preferred way of life. It is necessary to relinquish outdated patterns and beliefs that no longer benefit us and adopt novel modes of thinking and being. By embracing change, we paves the way for new opportunities and prospects for personal development and exploration.

Although uncertainty may induce unease, it is an inherent and indispensable component of the voyage. Trusting in oneself and the process is a prerequisite for embracing uncertainty, even when the trajectory ahead is hazy. It encourages us to embrace unease and venture into uncharted territories with bravery and inquisitiveness, recognizing that development frequently awaits beyond the threshold of uncertainty.

Adaptability is an extraordinarily valuable trait during the pursuit of minimalism, as it enables us to modify and pivot in an instant when conditions alter. Developing an adaptable mindset and embracing novelty enables individuals to enhance their resilience and resourcefulness when confronted with obstacles. By embracing the fluidity of life and relinquishing rigid expectations, we discover beauty and opportunity in the perpetual flux of existence.

As we endeavor to become the most advantageous versions of ourselves, transformation is the ultimate aim of the minimalist journey. Embracing change entails placing one's trust in the transformative process, knowing that every progressive step brings one closer to their true selves. By courageously and receptively embracing change, individuals unleash the capacity for personal development, satisfaction, and happiness.

Gaining Insight from Failures

It is unavoidable to encounter obstacles along the way, and the pursuit of minimalism is no exception. Conversely, setbacks can be reframed as valuable opportunities for learning and development, as opposed to disasters. Every obstacle that arises provides valuable knowledge regarding our aptitudes, deficiencies, and opportunities for growth, thereby strengthening our resolve and progress along the parsimonious path.

Resilience is among the most valuable teachings that can be gleaned from setbacks. Confronting challenges and setbacks directly fosters the development of interior fortitude and tenacity, thereby equipping individuals to confront forthcoming obstacles with enhanced assurance and poise. By viewing obstacles as chances to develop resilience, we can foster a positive outlook and resolute mindset when confronted with challenges.

In addition, setbacks offer insightful feedback that can guide subsequent actions and decisions. We can identify any patterns or behaviors that may have contributed to the outcome of a setback by analyzing the circumstances that preceded it. Having this self-awareness enables us to make more informed decisions and adjust our course accordingly, which ultimately results in increased achievement and satisfaction throughout our pursuit of minimalism.

Moreover, setbacks provide an opportunity for self-discovery and introspection. An analysis of our responses and reactions to obstacles can provide significant illumination regarding our values, priorities, and convictions. In the end, setbacks facilitate personal development by compelling us to confront our anxieties and limitations, thereby fostering an environment that is more empowering and resilient.

Ultimately, failures impart the value of perseverance and tenacity. When encountering obstacles or setbacks, there is often a temptation to surrender or stray from our intended objectives. Nevertheless, through the display of resilience and unwavering dedication to our overarching vision, we exhibit tenacity and perseverance, ultimately emerging from challenges more fortified and resilient.

By viewing obstacles as chances for development and progress, we can convert difficulties into pivotal moments along our pursuit of minimalism. Every obstacle provides significant insights into the virtues of resilience, self-awareness, and perseverance, which ultimately foster personal development and progress.

Commemorating Advances

Despite encountering obstacles and setbacks along the path to minimalism, it is critical to reflect and acknowledge the advancements that have been achieved. Each incremental progress, regardless of its magnitude, serves as evidence of our dedication, perseverance, and development. Through the act of recognizing and commemorating our accomplishments, we foster an atmosphere of appreciation, inspiration, and satisfaction that sustains our ongoing advancement along the minimalist trajectory.

Commemorating advancements enables us to recognize the diligence and commitment that have been devoted to streamlining our existence and striving towards our objectives. Experiencing validation and recognition for our endeavors enhances our self-assurance and motivation. We reinforce positive habits and behaviors and affirm our dedication to the minimalist way of life by devoting time to commemorate our accomplishments.

Further, commemorating advancements cultivates an attitude of appreciation for the copiousness that is already a part of our existence. We develop a mindset of affluence and gratitude by concentrating on our achievements rather than fixating on our shortcomings. Practicing gratitude broadens our perception of the splendor and advantages that indwell us, thereby augmenting our holistic sense of satisfaction and welfare.

Additionally, commemorating advancements provides encouragement and inspiration for the path that lies ahead. We obtain the confidence and impetus to continue approaching our objectives by contemplating how far we have come. Every accomplished milestone serves as a catalyst for motivation and self-empowerment, serving as a reminder of our potential for development and metamorphosis.

At last, the minimalist voyage is infused with a sense of joy and satisfaction when progress is commemorated. Engaging in this practice enables us to fully appreciate instances of triumph and attainment, deriving significance and intention from our endeavors. Adopting a celebratory mindset imbues one's voyage with optimism, positivity, and delight, thereby transforming the minimalist lifestyle into a genuinely gratifying and enlightening experience.

In summary, commemorating advancements is a fundamental practice throughout the pursuit of minimalism. Through the practice of recognizing our accomplishments, fostering an attitude of appreciation, and deriving pleasure from the process, we invigorate our drive, fortitude, and sense of satisfaction, thereby propelling us towards a more deliberate and uncomplicated lifestyle.

9

Conclusion: Living a Fulfilling Minimalist Life

Upon Grasping the Journey

In anticipation of the book's culmination and your progression towards adopting a minimalist lifestyle, pause momentarily to contemplate the path you have followed. Reflect upon the significant transformations that have occurred in your life, both internally and externally, since adopting the tenets of minimalism and purging your surroundings of debris.

Reflect on the advancements that have been achieved since the inception of this endeavor. Reflect upon the tangible belongings that you have relinquished, the routines that you have modified, and the cognitive transformations that have transpired throughout this process. Recognize the obstacles you have encountered and the fortitude you have exhibited in surmounting them. Applaud your triumphs, irrespective of their magnitude, and acknowledge the development and metamorphosis that you have experienced.

Assess the knowledge and insights that have been gained during the course of your minimalist voyage. Reflect upon the realizations that have been attained regarding one's self, values, and priorities. Consider the various ways in which the practice of minimalism has enhanced your life, promoting increased clarity, purpose, and satisfaction. How have the changes you have implemented affected your relationships, routines, and general state of being?

Upon introspection of your voyage, ensure that you identify the domains in which you continue to develop and progress. Acknowledge that minimalism is an ongoing journey of self-discovery and improvement, and not a fixed endpoint. In the coming days and weeks, reflect on how you can enhance the simplicity of your life, foster more meaningful connections, and ensure that your actions are in accordance with your personal values.

In essence, in the pursuit of a gratifying minimalist existence, introspection onto one's voyage facilitates the acquisition of insight, perspective, and gratitude. By recognizing one's personal growth and incorporating the knowledge gained, one can approach forthcoming endeavors with assurance, determination, and a positive outlook.

Accepting Gratitude

It is simple to forget about the bounties and abundance that envelop us amidst the frenzy of contemporary life. In the final moments of your pursuit of minimalist living, savor the moment and develop a profound sense of appreciation for everything that you possess. Adopting an attitude of gratitude as a guiding principle can significantly elevate one's life quality and sense of satisfaction.

Contemplating the elegance and simplicity of the minimalist way of life, recognize the opportunity and privilege it bestows upon you. Reflect upon the tranquility and independence that ensue from reducing one's possessions, and convey appreciation for the enhanced perception and understanding it imparts. Make an effort to be appreciative on a daily basis by devoting time to contemplation of the numerous and varied benefits that enhance your existence.

Appreciate those in your life who encourage and support you throughout your voyage. Acknowledge the affection, benevolence, and companionship that they bestow, and value the relationships that imbue your existence with happiness and significance. Foster an attitude of gratitude within your interpersonal connections by openly expressing your appreciation and benevolence towards those in your vicinity.

Embrace the simple pleasures of daily existence with gratitude. Embrace instances of aesthetic appeal, tranquility, and delight, such as an awe-inspiring sunset, a comforting cup of tea, or an intimate dialogue with a cherished individual. Adopt a mindset of gratitude that enables you to discover happiness and satisfaction in the current instant, irrespective of the situation.

Ultimately, convey appreciation for the expedition itself, encompassing the obstacles, regressions, and instances of development and metamorphosis. Acknowledge the fortitude, resolve, and bravery that have accompanied you on this journey, and commemorate the strides you have taken toward leading a more purposeful and gratifying existence.

Developing an attitude of gratitude can foster an increased degree of happiness, satisfaction, and contentment in one's existence. As one nears the culmination of their expedition into minimalist living, may gratitude serve as a guiding principle, casting a glow of grace, appreciation, and abundance upon the path ahead.

Resolving to Sustain Growth

Upon the culmination of your pursuit of minimalist living, it is critical to maintain a steadfast dedication to continuous development and advancement. A journey, not a destination, minimalism entails an ongoing progression of self-exploration, knowledge acquisition, and improvement. You can guarantee that your journey will continue to be dynamic, purposeful, and gratifying for many years by adopting this perspective.

Accept change as an inherent and indispensable component of the minimalist voyage. Be receptive to novel concepts, experiences, and viewpoints, and willing to confront your limitations by venturing beyond your comfort zone. One should embrace change as a chance for personal development and metamorphosis, having faith that every fresh phase will yield invaluable insights and lessons.

Continue to seek out opportunities for self-discovery, exploration, and learning as a personal challenge. Aim for personal development and growth in every aspect of your life, whether it be by attending workshops, reading, or participating in meaningful conversations. Maintain an open mind, curiosity, and inquisitiveness, and ceaseless pursuit of knowledge and comprehension.

Maintain steadfast dedication to your personal values and priorities while maneuvering through the intricacies of contemporary existence. Consistently evaluated your objectives, routines, and way of life decisions, and modify them accordingly in order to maintain congruence with your genuine identity. Bear in mind that the pursuit of minimalism is an exceedingly individual endeavor, and that no universal strategy applies. Maintain self-authenticity, rely on your intuition, and pay attention to your innermost counsel as you progress and develop.

Cultivate a mindset characterized by perseverance and resilience in the face of obstacles and adversity. Keep in mind that setbacks are learning and development opportunities, not failings. Blessing oneself with fortitude, resolve, and composure, one should confront challenges with the understanding that surmounting each impediment fortifies and fortifies one.

By dedicating oneself to ongoing development and transformation, one can guarantee that the pursuit of minimalist living remains dynamic, significant, and gratifying. On the journey towards a more deliberate and simplistic lifestyle, it is essential to maintain authenticity, embrace change, and actively pursue opportunities for personal growth and learning.

Cultivating Relationships

In the culmination of your pursuit of minimalist living, it is critical to place utmost importance on cultivating significant interpersonal relationships. Relationships are fundamental to achieving a sense of fulfillment in life; fostering genuine and substantial connections enhances our existence to an extraordinary degree. Invest effort into cultivating and fortifying the connections that you have with oneself, others, and the global community.

Develop a more profound connection with yourself initially. Invest time in self-reflection and introspection to gain a deeper understanding of yourself. Investigate your passions, values, and aspirations, and treat your needs and desires with compassion and generosity. Engage in activities that bring you pleasure and fulfillment, and prioritize self-care practices that nourish your body, mind, and spirit.

Make an effort to cultivate and support your interpersonal connections, be they with friends, family, or members of your community. Allocate time for substantive dialogues, communal experiences, and benevolent deeds that cultivate a sense of belonging and strengthen relationships. Develop understanding, compassion, and empathy in your interactions, and make quality time spent together a priority.

Make an effort to establish connections with the environment, be it through art, nature, or significant social issues. Alone in nature, luxuriate in its splendor and become engrossed in its serenity. Explore and appreciate works of literature, music, and art that elevate and inspire you, thereby cultivating a more profound admiration for the abundance and variety of human expression. Engage in volunteer work that is consistent with your personal values and interests, thereby effecting constructive transformation and effecting global impact.

Develop relationships with your community through volunteer work, participation in local events, and membership in organizations and groups that share your interests. Developing connections with individuals who share similar interests and goals can provide encouragement, motivation, and companionship throughout the pursuit of minimalist living.

Cultivating connections ultimately entails promoting a feeling of inclusion and interdependence in one's existence. You can enrich your life with affection, joy, and satisfaction by placing an emphasis on significant connections with yourself, others, and the world at large. As you near the end of your pursuit of minimalist living, may the connections you've formed serve as a wellspring of fortitude, encouragement, and motivation for the future.

Acceptance of the Journey

It is crucial that as you near the end of this book and your pursuit of minimalist living, you remain open to the continuous process of development, revelation, and metamorphosis. A journey to be cherished, minimalism is not a destination to be attained; rather, it is an ongoing process of self-discovery and development.

Accept life's fluctuations with a positive attitude, knowing that transformation is inescapable and viewing it as a chance to develop and rejuvenate. One should embrace the unpredictability and ambiguity of the future and have faith in their capacity to gracefully and resiliently navigate any obstacles and opportunities that may present themselves.

Commemorate the advancements achieved and the insights gained throughout the process. Commemorate the instances of lucidity, companionship, and elation that have profoundly enhanced your existence and expanded your comprehension of what it means to lead a life guided by intention and purpose.

Maintain an open mind toward new opportunities and experiences, remaining inquisitive, daring, and receptive to the awe-inspiring majesty of the world. Embrace the multitude and variety that comprise existence, relishing every moment with sincerity and admiration.

Ultimately, wholeheartedly Embrace the Journey—Its turbulence and success, obstacles and successes, and fluctuations. Acknowledge and embrace the journey of self-exploration and development, for each stride you undertake brings you one step closer to living a life congruent with your principles, interests, and life's mission.

As you near the culmination of your pursuit of minimalist living, welcome the journey with a receptive attitude and a sense of inquisitiveness, appreciation, and amazement. One can continuously evolve and develop by embracing the voyage; in doing so, they will discover joy and satisfaction in the ongoing process of self-transformation and exploration.